Arunachalam Kumar

Biped Stance & Stride

Arunachalam Kumar

Biped Stance & Stride

Origin & Evolution Of Orthograde Posture & Gait

LAP LAMBERT Academic Publishing

Impressum / Imprint

Bibliografische Information der Deutschen Nationalbibliothek: Die Deutsche Nationalbibliothek verzeichnet diese Publikation in der Deutschen Nationalbibliografie; detaillierte bibliografische Daten sind im Internet über http://dnb.d-nb.de abrufbar.

Alle in diesem Buch genannten Marken und Produktnamen unterliegen warenzeichen-, marken- oder patentrechtlichem Schutz bzw. sind Warenzeichen oder eingetragene Warenzeichen der jeweiligen Inhaber. Die Wiedergabe von Marken, Produktnamen, Gebrauchsnamen, Handelsnamen, Warenbezeichnungen u.s.w. in diesem Werk berechtigt auch ohne besondere Kennzeichnung nicht zu der Annahme, dass solche Namen im Sinne der Warenzeichen- und Markenschutzgesetzgebung als frei zu betrachten wären und daher von jedermann benutzt werden dürften.

Bibliographic information published by the Deutsche Nationalbibliothek: The Deutsche Nationalbibliothek lists this publication in the Deutsche Nationalbibliografie; detailed bibliographic data are available in the Internet at http://dnb.d-nb.de.

Any brand names and product names mentioned in this book are subject to trademark, brand or patent protection and are trademarks or registered trademarks of their respective holders. The use of brand names, product names, common names, trade names, product descriptions etc. even without a particular marking in this works is in no way to be construed to mean that such names may be regarded as unrestricted in respect of trademark and brand protection legislation and could thus be used by anyone.

Coverbild / Cover image: www.ingimage.com

Verlag / Publisher:
LAP LAMBERT Academic Publishing
ist ein Imprint der / is a trademark of
AV Akademikerverlag GmbH & Co. KG
Heinrich-Böcking-Str. 6-8, 66121 Saarbrücken, Deutschland / Germany
Email: info@lap-publishing.com

Herstellung: siehe letzte Seite /
Printed at: see last page
ISBN: 978-3-659-44121-9

CONTENTS

1

Location of locomotor appendages

Evolution is characterized by two attributes: one is to find sustenance for life and the other, the need to multiply. Any or all changes in shape, size, cerebration and adaptations are engendered by need to meet these primary requirements and the need to acquire higher efficiency in finding mate or manna. Towards achieving these ends, locomotion as an adjunct aid has evolved as a powerful tool. Try pulling off a suckling piglet or pup from the dam's teats. The suckling infant grips the mammary gland with all its infantile might using the power of its clenched gum. In effect, the grip mimics a 'towards gland' movement against an 'away from gland' yank direction. That the mouth and its parts do play an imperceptible but definitely identifiable role in 'limb' activity is evidenced by the atavistic 'oro-facial reflex' seen during dexterous manual (digital) movements. Oro-facial reflex moments are seen to increase proportional to acuity of dexterity employed by the hand.

It would not be erroneous to infer that, the mouth is probably an archaic primary locomotor appendage, regressing in its scope and range over the eons of evolution where limbs (fore and hind) took over the function of engendering mobility. One of more peculiar observations is the progressive and gradual caudal locus shift of appendages that engineer locomotion. The more primitive the form of life, the more cranial is the appendage that initiates movement.

Invertebrates kick-start mobility using their mouth parts as anchoring mechanisms that help drag themselves forwards. Classically, the earthworm and leech are examples where mouth plays a very crucial role in movement. Fish use apparatuses like gills or fins and early reptiles use rudimentary pectoral accruements. The metamorphosis of the aquatic tadpole into a quadruped amphibian appears to confirm this hypothesis. Tadpoles anchor themselves onto blades of grass or weed with their mouth to brace themselves against currents using. Their fixing is a form of paradoxical movement against the current direction. Such paradoxical locomotion is seen often in many species, even terrestrial ones.

The cranio-caudal displacement of primary mechanisms that help mobility during the various stages of tadpole to frog development will show that when an early tadpole the amphibian uses its mouth to anchor itself to a blade or stalk to anchor itself against a flowing current (a paradoxical propulsion) – it graduates to using pectoral fin like appendages – thence to forelimbs, then it develops hind limbs as additions. The adult frog primarily depends on catapulting itself onwards relying mainly on the strength and power of its hind limbs. Aves depend heavily on the fore limb power to move fly, the hind limbs are merely adjuncts that aid the forelimb (modified into wings) to augment and refine aerial movement.

The mouth parts as a whole, lips, teeth, gums, tongue included, can and do play a 'grip or grasp' role in steadying, itself a paradoxical propulsive action. While the drafting of the oral accruements into performance of activities, as adjunct or as replacement for limb participation is rather commonplace and in lower life forms, such as hydra, leeches and caterpillars and other invertebrates using 'looping', oral activation as part of limb performance is also observed in many vertebrates. Animals like elephants or rhinoceroses, use their elongated upper lip as 'handy' appendages – the usage being extreme in elephants, in whom the extension of the median nasal process - philtrum upper lip complex becomes a dependable and much used prehensile 'limb'; In fact, the Hindi term for elephant is 'haathi' from' haath' – hand.

Among the mammalians, man alone, has developed into dependence on highly evolved hind limbs (legs) for movement. Even in man, the most extreme end of his foot, the great toe is the primary generator of bipedal gait.

What is seen from the examples cited is that from the lowest forms of life, as one goes up the evolutionary tree – the apparatuses and appendages that help it move – show a distinct tendency to shift from head to tail end: a cranio-caudal displacement of primary and principal locomotor apparatuses and bio-mechanisms. It is a scientific curio worth dwelling on. That one can even place a life form into its slot in the evolutionary scale tree merely by noting the position of its propulsive mechanical apparatuses: The more head-ward propulsive appendages are, the more primitive the life form is, and vice versa.

It has been observed that in some animals, using mouth / nose / tail as accruements that can aid or initiate movement: yet it would seem strange to learn that the ability use mouth parts are adjuncts to movement. In fact as described elsewhere it is indeed so. The description of the atavistic oro-facial reflex is example of how the mouth, involuntarily, plays a role.

Years of observation over large populations have reinforced my surmise that a hitherto unnoticed facial reaction is a legacy of atavism. The higher the degree of digital dexterity involved in the performance of manual tasks, the more striking is the involuntary reaction of orofacial muscles to the level of concentration the task requires. Watch a volunteer thread a needle; the individual either purses his lips, or contorts his mouth, or licks his lips, or bites his tongue tip; an orofacial-lingual response to manual work?

As this is a very widespread and universally human response, it must have either a functional or atavistic basis, if not so. In quadrupeds, simians specially, the mouth or its component parts, the teeth, lips or tongue, are used as adjuncts to bimanual work. The use of oral appendages as adjunct aids in performance of manual tasks certainly makes, tearing, ripping, or carrying food or material.

Is the involuntary reaction of facial grimace, twitch, wetting, or clenching the jaw, a physiological atavistic trait carried over into the higher mammal? How does the contraction of orbicularis oris or the action of genioglossus muscle influence the performance of task at 'hand'?

There is no obvious correlation or between the disparate muscular masses, the direct use of the hand lumbricals to perform concentrated manual chore, and the simultaneous, but, indirect oro-facial muscular action of the mouth and tongue. The muscle groups involved (in hand and of mouth) are neither contiguous nor congruous or complementary, yet they occur together.

It is inferred that the digito-oro-facial-lingual response to performance of manual work requiring concentrated effort is an un-reported evolutionary vestige and a classic, but odd, non-anatomical vestige of atavism.

Of similar genre is the tripping over or falling seen in bipeds. The kinetics of biped gait make the human unstable. The tendency to fall is very inherent to movement on two supports (legs). But observe the fall: it is always forwards – almost never

5

backwards. Whenever a man trips, he stumbles forwards – the reflex direction of fall enables him to quickly support his falling weight on his outstretched hands (forelimbs). This protective reflex mechanism is inborn.

2

How animals move

Gait, quadruped or biped has much mystery to it. The trials and course correction evolution has engendered in perfecting propulsive mechanisms and apparatuses have been subject to much analysis and argument among researchers of evolutionary biology.

Why do some birds hop while some walk? Why does an ape walk on its knuckles? How did the anthropoid ape develop biped gait? Why do bears or camels take strides using a single side of their body parts, one half after another. That is both right sided fore and hind limbs act in concert, then the process is followed by the other, the left side doing the same. A lumbering, rolling-rocking side to side gait!

Observe a quadruped walk across a low hurdle or ledge. It takes one forelimb after another to get over the rise, then amazingly doesn't repeat the same one after another maneuver with its hind limbs – instead it leaps or hops this time, using both its rear legs, in unison.

Though seemingly trivial, this climbing over a hurdle or step mechanism bears much intrigue. In fact, it may well be cerebral. The animal has eyes which guide it front two limbs carefully one after another to overcome the ledge – then, once the template of the height to be overcome and the muscular power required gets registered in its brain – the higher centers of the cerebrum now take over and simplifies the earlier forelimb activity, this time perfecting bipedal hind limb to perform in coordinated synchrony.

Ground hugging terrestrial movement, slither, is a limbless advance using scales. Serpents move in three forms, rectilinear, curvilinear (sinuous) or 'concertina'. Some can sidle sideways, lifting parts of their lengths off the ground level.

One of the more striking observations has been that the rat snake moves much faster than the cobra. The logic behind the need for speed could be that it is less feared and therefore more vulnerable. The cobra by contrast slithers slower than the rat snake – it need not hurry, it can defend itself quite effectively when cornered.

Snakes possess two types of locomotion. Preferentially, constrictors and their ilk perform 'rectilinear' progression while most others use 'curvilinear' movement. The vertebral column of the constrictors does not swing one way and another. Though the vertebral surfaces of both species snakes are 'procoelous', they choose to deploy different modes of mobility. Cobras cover less distance than rat snakes during a given time period: The question is, despite being as agile and alert as the rat snake, why does the cobra cover less ground? (apart from the reason given earlier).

My observations show that the rat snake swings less from side to side: its spinal column shifts less from the axis than it does in the cobra. The cobra's movement shows that its loops are smaller, but deeper. The measure of the amplitude of shift from the axis is more in the cobra than in the rat snake. The extra deep loops (curves) slows the cobra considerably

Even from a fair distance I have been able to identify (with reasonably confident rate of accuracy) either of the two species of snakes just by observing the 'sinuousness' of their backbones and speed of their progression.

Observe a quadruped walk across a low hurdle or ledge. It takes one forelimb after another to get over the rise, then amazingly doesn't repeat the same one after another maneuver with its hind limbs – instead it leaps or hops this time, using both its rear legs, in unison.

Though seemingly trivial, this climbing over a hurdle or step mechanism bears much intrigue. In fact, it may well be cerebral. The animal has eyes which guide it front two limbs carefully one after another to overcome the ledge – then, once the template of the height to be overcome and the muscular power required gets registered in its brain – the higher centers of the cerebrum now take over and simplifies the earlier forelimb activity, this time perfecting bipedal hind limb to perform in coordinated synchrony.

Gait, quadruped or biped has much mystery to it. The trials and course correction evolution has engendered in perfecting propulsive mechanisms and apparatuses have been subject to much analysis and argument among researchers of evolutionary biology.

Trot, gallop, strut, hop, slide, stride, bound, leap, lope, roll, tumble, slither, and knuckle-walking are terms used to define types of terrestrial locomotion in quadrupeds. Another odd term is pronging. Each term, by definition is specific to one or more species and describes one particular mode of progression. Brachiating, scaling, climbing, flying, gliding, hovering, soaring describe movement through air or trees, swimming, skimming, wadding, treading, paddling are methods used when water is the medium.

3

The bipedal bird

One of the more intriguing questions in avian locomotion is why some birds, when on ground, choose to hop while others prefer walking. Biped gait is common to birds as well as the most evolved among mammals, man. Observations made show that, choice of gait in birds is determined by a remote factor – the range and extent of neck mobility. The wider the gamut of cervical mobility, the wider is the 'field of vision' available. Cervical movement capability is perhaps the single most deterministic factor in the bird's choice of terrestrial gait.

One of the earliest bipeds to survive to modern era, are birds. Birds are unique in that many species among them have capability of flying in air, walking on land and swimming in water. The talent to exploit all three mediums, air, land and water for mobility makes birds occupy special in the evolutionary tree.

The biped gait in birds has thrown up variants. While do some birds walk while some others hop? This rather simple question throws up quite interesting and debatable answers. This brief article proposes that extra mobility of neck produced by wider cervical intervertebral articular range, in turn causes the bird to augment its visual range, which in turn allows the bird to progress slowly step by step. In birds with limited neck movement (reduced cervical intervertbral articular capacity) the biped gait is modified into hopping instead of striding. Hopping allows such birds to pivot round or turn abruptly. In essence, the choice of gait, hopping or walking, is determined by visual field – which in turn is controlled by mobility range of neck .Observations on biped mobility on birds and their locomotion reveal that, generally smaller birds hop while larger ones stride, strut or walk. Many theories and hypotheses float around the word of ornithology and kinematics on the how and why of avian locomotion.

a) Raptors (kites, eagles, hawks, owls) and other such birds, hop and strut far less than their arboreal and more terrestrial cousins, the passerines.

b) Arboreal and terrestrial, or low flying birds ground hop and walk more than the hi-fliers or nocturnal cousins

c) Birds that are endowed with a better degree of cervical (neck) vertebral rotation hop less. That is, birds that have limited swivel of neck (up to 180 or less) hop more and more frequently than the birds that can rotate their heads through a much wider arc. Some birds have a complete or nearly complete 360-degree field of view. Birds such as owls are gifted with nearly 270 plus range of side to side swivel of neck vertebrae. The ability to rotate the head and increase field of vision to almost full circle range, makes the birds on alert to approaching danger – the talent to spot peril early, gives them the confidence to progress one step at a time (walk).Owls possess twice the number of cervical vertebrae, fourteen. The extra articulations in the cervix allows for more efficiency and fluidity (and range) in neck mobility.

Birds also have more cervical vertebrae than many other animals; most have a highly flexible neck consisting of 13-25 vertebrae. Similar too is the gait long necked birds and raptors. In anatomical terms, the intervertebral cervical joints have wider articular surfaces of the plane / condlylar type in birds that soar, hover, or nocturnal. These birds, hypothetically at least, being gifted with a wider eye view and range of vision, thanks to an efficient cervical mobility, require less need to hop, twist and turn their whole bodies to visualize a wider field. They end up

11

having to use their legs for walking. In less mobile necked birds, hopping, in of lieu striding, allows shift of range and focus in field of vision in continuously.

d) The natural processes of adaptation has perhaps given birds that strut and hop less with better cervical articular vertebral inputs, and vice versa, birds that can better hop, jump, strut and perch, need less efficiency in head rotation and mobility - the range and axis of movement of the cervical intervertebral joints accentuating or diminishing range of field of vision.

Prey species, like pigeons and robins, usually have a very wide field of view because they need to see danger coming from any direction. To achieve this most of their vision is monocular, like our peripheral vision, with only a narrow angle of binocular vision with good depth perception

A pigeon can see nearly 360 around its head, a real advantage when avoiding a peregrine. It's so important for birds to see what's coming, that some prey species can even move each eye independently! Research into visual range and peripheral vision in some waders conclude that neck positioning plays a major role in success in foraging.

Predator species usually have a narrower field of view because they need to have good depth perception in order to capture prey. The owl's field of view is more like ours with a wide area of binocular vision and narrow bands of peripheral, monocular vision on either side. Peregrines have fields of view similar to owls. The chicken and the pigeon are two good examples of this. Such birds must judge distance by moving their heads and viewing an object with each eye independently, deducing from the displacement how far away the object must be.

The possibility of that neck mobility and visual ranges could be inter-dependent and complement type of gait used has not been thought of yet. Birds do not possess well developed muscles for eyeball movement they rely on their ability to maneuver their head and neck for good visualization of objects.

As these observations and conclusions derived are conjectural, speculative and hypothetical, the entire question of biomechanics and of neck as having bearing on bipedal kinetics may require a much deeper probe. Perimetrical visual analysis and collation of data on orbital fields in passerines, perchers, raptors and predators should aid in clarifying issues to some extent.

Note:

Rarely does biology repeat a failed experiment. Bipedalism as mode of terrestrial locomotion was given up as an evolution improved model: a reversion to quadruped gait was result of this seemingly 'failed' experiment. Yet, eons and millennia later, evolution picks up the 'biped' model again, introducing it for one more run among australopithecine.

4

Knuckle walking

Erect posture and bipedalism as a preferred mode for life and locomotion are uniquely human traits. Much debate has centered round the origins, time and sequence of the hind-limb weight support and propulsion characteristic, a hominid attribute. In my line of work, anatomy, I have probed a little bit on the biomechanics of the pollex-index 'opposition' (it must be recalled here that the liberation of the pollex (thumb) and the conversion of the first carpometacarpal joint from a condylar into a saddle, enabled the thumb to be opposed to the index). The free-ing of the forelimbs into performance of higher, more compulsive, and educated tasks from its hitherto chore of supporting body weight and mobility, is claimed to be the cornerstone of bipedalism, and thence from into the explosion of cerebration that led to the genesis of bipeds into rational homos.

What yet remains un-probed is, why or how the forelimb skeletal architecture modified into a need and functionally related instrument. Going further back into the world of higher apes, the gorillas, one observes that locomotion is essentially a quadruped activity, but oddly, the forelimb in gorilla, is not held 'paw down', but backward. That is, the animal is a knuckle walker, supporting its weight on the knuckles of the front legs. The digits are flexed and curled inwards, the paw (palmar) pads are held protected with the limb terminating into a fisted hand-paw. Why so, And so abruptly at that did the forelimb turn inwards into a clenched fist. Why, when every quadruped walked on paw pads, did the gorilla decide to walk on knuckles?

The change in kinematics and biomechanics of the forelimb does engender debate. Did the phalanges elongate and lengthen? Did the digits become arachnoid? Was

14

walking on the front paw now more hazardous and maiming to the now elongated spindly digits? Were the fingertips and nails becoming too injury-prone compromising the efficiency of non-locomotor functions. Did anyone or all these factors make the evolving ape to turn its digits inwards?

Was the higher induced to flex its finger tips to protect them from injuries (avulsion of nail, pulp infections etc) Flexion is a universally acknowledged action for protection. Every animal, including an invertebrate curls itself into a posture of complete flexion when sensing danger. Man too does so, even in his foetal in-utero existence. That being so, with the forelimb digital phalanges lengthening and becoming more prone to knocks and injury, the gorilla and other late brachiators, maybe sought to guard their new anatomically delicate appendages and protect their evolutionary acquisitions – they perhaps did this – by curling (flexing) them inwards. Now walking had to be done on knuckles, not on the fore-foot pads. It may be of some interest to note that the dorsal (knuckle) surfaces of the inter-phalangeal joints are protected by a dense fascia that caps the fingers precisely and right on the joint capsules. The dorsal digital expansion serves protects the joint on its knuckles – no such fascial modification is found on the flexor (palmar) surface of the very same joints – probably explaining why it was wiser and more prudent to use the knuckle instead of the foot pad as weight supporting accruements.

The question now arises, did this shift over to palmar flexion, and the biomechanics of opposition evolution go hand in hand, or not? If not, and knuckle supported mobility was prelude to opposition, then such walkers indeed form a vital link in evolution of human erect posture and gait – knuckle walking should form the first link in the chain that led to bipedalism. Were the gorilla and great ape front paw evolving into a more complex and kinetically efficient structure?

Was this the prelude to the liberation of the thumb? Is knuckle walking the key to understanding the sequences and events leading to cerebral growth?

Whatever the debate, the fact remains, knuckle walk as a preferred mode of weight bearing and locomotion has too long been looked at as a purely biomechanical means of propulsion: it is time physical anthropologists, kinesiologists and evolutionary biologists reviewed the signal and heraldic role the simple flexion of the fore limb phalanges has played in the final evolution of a hominin with an opposable thumb and a biomechanically efficient bipedal stride and stance.

5

The lacrimal apparatus

In our desperate need to find answers we often rely on skeletal remains to tell their tales of origin and fate. Physical anthropologists have too long concentrated on ostoelogical factors to draw conclusions or propose newer theories on the origins of the man.

Today, science, delving deep into genetics and other nascent specialties, has made anthropological studies easier, and perhaps more reliable. Yet, one often wonders, whether we are ignoring any telltale evidences of evolution, often manifest in us and around us. In my line of work, as a teacher of human anatomy to medical students, I have often stumbled upon an odd anatomical feature or two that seemed quite out of place in the utopian functional design and efficiency of the highest form of evolution, man. Take for example, the lachrymal (lacrimal) apparatus…

Some years ago, observing my pet dog, attempt to dislodge a foreign body from it's own eye, I saw, fascinated, a unique maneuver that promptly expelled the offending alien particle. The dog, just used its front paw to shut the edge of one side of its nose and nostril, and induced a sneeze, which in turn, expelled the foreign body. Intrigued, I experimented again and again with the animal and in some others too and then on my friends (all medical students). In every case, shutting of the contralateral nostril (the left, if the foreign body is in the right eye), and inducting a sneeze, dislodged any superficially located particle. So effective and noninvasive was the procedure, that I even reported it in a medical journal as a simple first aid procedure

Over the years, I have off and on recommended the procedure even in patients with chronic dachrocystitis and epiphora. The maneuver repeated over a time, clears the lacrimal ducts and restores their patency, often non-surgically. Now what has all this got to do with evolution you may wonder? It does, I think.

I have since dissected the lachrymal sac in a number of human cadavers and studied them grossly as well as microscopically. The apparatus consists of two minute canals, which originate at the upper and lower lid's medial edge. Each canal then takes an abrupt angulation, to converge towards its fellow duct. Here they open into a fusiform sac, which in turn, open ended (bottomless, except for a flap of mucous membrane) caudally to open directly into the lateral wall of the nasal cavity. The ducts convey secretions produced by the lacrimal gland, which bathes the corneal surface of our eye. The secretion is an oil-watery saline, which acts as a moisturizer and sterilizes the exposed eye surface.

Physiologically, in man at least, the gland has little other function, excepting as an ineffective aid to excretion of salts. The question is, why would nature design such a complicated apparatus for something which performs so little, function wise? Nature does not condone waste in investment. Is the lacrimal sac performing some other role in man? For that, the answer is found in the quadrupeds, as I found in my dog.

So what is the role of the sac? A dilated balloon, made up of fibro-elastic tissue: Elastic? Why? Why should the sac want to recoil? from what? for what?

The spent secretions of the eye are transported by the canals into the sac where it pools up, wherefrom it percolates into the nose to dry up with the warmth of the inspired air. But why is nature storing this waste? A few droplets of lacrimal secretion is held within each sac, which has a simple flap valve at its lower end (an ineffective valve at that!) Now let me assume I am a dog (or a donkey maybe, as many of you would be tempted to suggest!). I have this irritating particle that flew into my eye, so, I presto, shut my left nostril, sneeze....and in the process increase my intranasal pressure, which increase flips open the valve at the caudal end of the sac, which then is subject to some intense reverse pressure, reacting to the stress by violently contracting its elastic components. This contraction shuts the valve, and forces the sac stored lacrimal fluid back along the ducts, in a reverse flow. The fluid now jets out off the punctae at the medial edges of the eyelid...the jet stream of saline washes across the cornea like a windscreen wiper and flushes out the foreign body from the eye. So that's the function of the lacrimal apparatus! Then why isn't man using the maneuver himself? Hmmm.. ...That is because he's turned biped!!

What is bipedalism doing here?

The lacrimal apparatus's efficiency is severely compromised by our erect posture and the reverse pressure required by man to flush back fluid from his sac up the eye is enormous and strenuous: But in a quadruped, a cinch! The sac lies at an easy sloping antigravity level, a small sniff or sneeze does the trick; in us, we need to try harder, but it works. Try sniffing some snuff, and watch how forcefully you sneeze, and how so much fluid gushes and brims your eye. Try with one nostril shut if you must.

So what does all this show? That may be bipedalism has not only changed the way eye things foreign, but has also changed the way we deal with foreign bodies in the eye. In our evolutionary hurry to go biped, we have lost out a very important and useful function of one of our old friends, the lacrimal sac. Now the poor sac, is just used to fill excess tears of a sobbing session.

What is the fate of the gland and sac now? Will it regress or become atavistic in years to come and go the way of our appendix or caudal appendage? I sincerely hope that we rediscover the potential of the lacrimal gland and its original function, and use a sneeze to expel any foreign body…and thus pay our dues to the machinations of evolutionary compromise. If not, R.I.P., Lacrimal Apparatus, Sac & Gland, I will miss you. Sob, sob, sniff, sniff. If you have tears, prepare to shed them now.

6

Universal flexion

Watch the 'mum to be' walk; Ungainly, tipping over gait, with the third trimester foetus pushing against her anterior abdominal wall, stretching the muscles to tautness. Look at her as she carefully weaves her way in that insanely narrow aisle at the supermarket, careful mum, that shopper yonder seems to be in haste as she careens ahead erratically towards her. Then just in the nick of time, a collision is averted, a deft side-step….and the oncoming peril is averted. It is not the evasive side-stepping maneuver of the mum to be that gets me curious, it is another instinctive action she takes to protect her unborn baby. She has hastily removed both her hands from the shopping cart, and folded her elbows defensively on her abdomen, her wrists flex and digits curl.

Flexion is a natural mechanism, the first line of defense against perceived dangers. Watch how the caterpillar curls itself, or that pangolin; or any quadruped for that matter. Universal flexion, every joint in flexion, is used to protect every vital organ in the abdomen, pelvis, or thorax, against assault. Why even the growing foetus in that mums womb, is in a position of universal flexion. But our 'mum to be' just has to make do with just two forearms flexed against her abdomen as her only line of defence. Ever wondered why?

The answer is evolution. With the emergence of Homo erectus, the additional flexion-induced protective shield available from the two lower limbs has been lost to the bipedal human. Were she still a quadruped, sighting the oncoming peril at the mall, our mum would have squatted, or crouched, and drawn her knees up close, in complete flexion along with the hip, the vertebral column itself would have flexed through contraction of the abdominal recti…but now, she just has to stand erect, the product of seven months of gestation, exposed to any, or all elements that threaten frontally.

I have discussed how I thought about the human lacrimal gland, and more particularly the apparatus appended to it, was slowly becoming functionally insignificant thanks to erect posture and our two- legged mobility attribute. The question I raise now is, could not the partial loss of protective flexion, with specific reference to the 'mum to be' analogy cited, be wholly attributed to the acquisition of bipedal gait and erect posture? Is the modern Mrs. Eve paying the price for a decision her ancestor, Mrs. Lucy took three million years ago, to move on in life, and up the evolutionary ladder, on two, not four limbs?

Should another tear ready to be shed for 'bipedalism'? Is the time tested reflex of 'universal flexion' being shoved out of our lives? Evolution took away my appendix, my platysma, my pyramidalis, and my auricular muscles.. It docked my tail. It has compromised the capabilities and range of flexion in the gravid human female…what next? Pardon me mate, I must shed some tears, right away, for turning biped and erect. Pass another tissue please…. quick, quick before evolution deletes even that tear shedding function of my lacrimals totally.

7

Squatting facets

As a professional human anatomist my work involves close handling and interface with osteology. One day, as I squatted to reach for a specimen from the bottom shelf of the departmental museum cupboard, it struck me that the position I was in, was uncannily stable. That an 'unlocked' knee could support or transmit the entire human weight, without fatigue, over long periods of time is against the dictates of biomechanical efficiency. Yet Asians can squat, oblivious to time, with nary a sweat bead of tiredness. How come?

Text books of anatomy describing kinetics of joints do mention some details on movement limitation in joints, but fail to cite that a very vital component of joint mobility range is the physical abutment of bone against bone (soft tissue is only a secondary factor). That is, the elbow cannot be hyperextended only because the olecranon of the ulna, fits so completely and fully into its eponymous fossa on the back of the humerus, that no further movement is possible. This juxtapositioning of articulating bones limits hypermobility in joints. Now if a similar case is made out for the knee, complete flexion, as done during squatting, should lead to a bone to bone impaction of the femur with tibia. This alone will relieve the muscles from acting their potential out in holding up their antigravity activity and tiring out. Then we, the Asiatic should have some osteological marker on the involved bones, tibia and femur, exactly at the point where these two bones grind to a halt against each other during complete flexion - and there it was - a small depression above the adductor tubercle of the femur that fitted perfectly with the posterior rim of the medial condyle of the tibia. The squatting facet of the femur!

Probably common to most squatters, but absent in non-squatters the femoral facet could aid in physical anthropological studies especially in forensic medicine, and in skeletal identifications during mass disasters. A spin off from this observation was a theory that I have often mulled over, but have no scholarship or confidence to back up. Primitive man was a squatter, and squatting, that is sitting on ones haunches, is a purely bipedal trait. Quadrupeds cannot squat, they need to support their ischial tuberosities on the ground to complete the kinematic chain that now distributes their own body weight along four points, two ischia and two feet (hind legs).

If my premise is reasonable, then we arrive at another interesting deduction. If habitual squatters and only bipeds have the femoral squatting facet, then logically the first bipeds, the non-brachiating proto-hominids or australopithecines should show the femoral facet. Do they?

I would look for such evidence to support any contention that Lucy stood on two legs and propelled herself bipedally. Of course, changes do occur in bipeds in the shape and tilt of the pelvis, and in various other skeletal features that support bipedal propulsion, but the presence or absence of the femoral squatting facet should be an adjunct piece of evidence to support such a view. Does the A. ardi femur have such a facet? I wonder? If present, Lucy, walked; if not, maybe not.

Joint movements have limitations in the range of movement: usually, the extent to which the articular surfaces juxtapose each other in a joint, movement is possible. Described also is the fact that when, say the elbow is flexed, despite there being an additional few square millimeters available for movement, the joints stop short: the halt in range is brought about by the abutment of muscle masses of the forearm and arm. So too, deposition of adipose tissue (fat) can limit joint movement.

There is yet another factor not cited in books or research: that is a joint's movement can be halted by bone abutting bone; when this happens the points of contact form facets, some of which may even go on to become synovial joints by themselves – the uncovertebral joint is one such. Usually facets so formed are seen in the lower limb skeletal elements. The so called 'squatting facets' created through the posture of squatting on the haunches, are seen in the upper and lower ends of the femur, lower end of tibia and neck of talus.

8

Conjectures

To turn bipedal was a choice anthropoid the higher apes made in exchange of some sacrifices. A quadruped stride and leap covers far greater distance than the biped stride any human can. Speed too had to be compromised. Most large four-legged animals lope faster than the fastest man. For the hunter-gatherer living in hard times, facing slim odds of survival in a wild and violent world, the option to go biped was a hugely risky one.

Consider the case of the earlier biped product of evolution, the avian. Birds too turned to biped mobility – yet, had to quickly learn to outpace competition or enemy by developing the once terrestrial locomotor aid, the forelimb, into the wing. Mastery over flight gave birds such a major advantage, that they survive till today: the only specimen in the evolutionary tree to conquer all three elemental mediums – terrestrial, aerial and aquatic – no other product of nature has this ability. Excepting birds, all higher evolutionary forms reverted to quadruped gait.

A similar experiment nature made is with bats: it is the only mammal that can fly. Yet, it has to sacrifice, almost completely, its ability of move on its two hind limbs, almost vestiges functionally. In the marsupials, kangaroos and wallabies, bipedal gait has modified to a hopping one, the forelimbs being reduced, both in size and function. Hopping as an exclusive mode of gait did not find much foothold, remaining restricted to a few isolated animals.

Coming back to the anthropoid apes and early proto hominids found that despite a compromise in speed and covered distance by choosing the option to prefer biped progression, the advantages accruing to the species as a whole and individual in particular was well worth the choice. Among the pluses touched and discussed upon by evolutionary biologists and physical anthropologists are:

1. Standing and moving in erect posture reduces surface area exposed directly to sun (and heat)

2. By liberating the forelimbs from participation in locomotion, the early biped found multiple applications and uses for the forepaws and limbs.

3. The freeing of the forelimb, in fact, in turn is said to have led to an explosion in cerebration – the brain now had the tool, the hands and was perforce to think of applications, new usages and methods: the thought process and ingenuity of the brain in redeploying the forelimbs is considered to be one of the significant catalysts for cerebral size increase. The early biped could now use hands and forelimbs to carry, clutch or fight.

4. The erect posture, adjunct to development bipedal gat, allowed the anthropoid ape to have a clearer view of their surroundings. The extra height the head was now carried permitted range of vision to increase substantially

5. By shifting the long axis of their bodies from the quadruped longitudinal to vertical, biped man and his erect posture, gained functional efficiency in their cervical vertebral articular capabilities. Early man's inter-vertebral joints could now be rotated to a greater range in the new axis.

6. With erect posture, the overhead reach of the forelimbs (hands) increased dramatically: an advantage that could be exploited for holding on to branches, climbing or plucking.

7. A unique attribute of biped gait is the development of the skill to side-step. Reflex sidestepping has numerous advantages. Quadrupeds can only hop / leap / spring side-ward, not sidestep.

8. Energy expended: There are some controversial debates on whether biped gait, uses almost the more, less or same energy as in quadruped. Yet there is dispute in the fact that, standing erect locks the knee joints further reducing energy consumption by liberating the lower limb musculature from need to hold up body weight. The locked knee converts the lower limb in to an osteological pillar needing little or no muscular truss or support.

9. A less obvious but significant advantage accruing in choice of bipedalism as preferred mode of locomotion is that the now free hands can (and do) at times of confrontation or combat with frontal approaching assault or danger, move to cover the face, head and neck. When under attack, the victim involuntarily masks his head – protectively.

10. One of the peculiar advantages of bipedal gait is the acquisition of ability to walk backwards. A few quadrupeds do so to, but only over a few strides or short distances – like when backing up to gain strike strength like in head-butting rams. Or when cringing in fright – a deer from a snake.

Man however has refined the art of striding backwards – he can and does back away with ease. The 'edge' in mobility is demonstrated when confronting danger – walking backwards slowly while facing the enemy (say a wild animal) not only distances you from peril and risk, but also allows one to keeping eyes focused on the attacker and is movements.

Humans can not only can walk but also run backwards, in fact even leap backwards. This talent was brought to light by a mechanical engineer, who taught himself and the world how one could leap backwards by taking better mechanical advantage of the thigh musculature – in fact, so successful was his attempt, that right from its debut date to today, every gold medal winner in high jump has used the backward leap, the 'Fosbury flop' (so named after the enterprising athlete engineer)

Another unexpected spin-off in opting for bipedalism and erect posture was that that the two legged posture and mobility enabled weights / loads to be carried on the head. No other animal, apart from the human, can carry head-loads. Just by using one hand to support the load from toppling, man can walk or run, keeping the other hand free – more importantly, experienced head-load carriers do not use hands at all. Once firmly placed and balanced atop the skull, the human can carry quite heavy weights even without the help of hands. The advantage this new skill gave to early man must have been huge: imagine being able to carry something without using hands! Erect posture and biped locomotion enabled man to carry a child, riding astride the shoulders; this mode of toting kids astride shoulders, is even now widely prevalent across all cultures and geographical locales and even seen in among apes.

A less obvious but significant advantage accruing in choice of bipedalism as preferred mode of locomotion, is that the now-free hands can (and do) at times of confrontation or combat with frontal approaching assault or danger, move protectively to cover the face, head and neck. When under attack, the victim involuntarily masks his head.

The disadvantages of biped gait:

1. Reduction in speed. The stride length is far less in bipeds than in quadrupeds. Length can certainly be increased considerably by running, but the preferred mode of locomotion is walking

2. Reduction in stride lengths

3. Frontal exposure to enemy and danger

4. Increased load, stress and strain on the vertebral column, the pelvis and post pelvic elements

5. Increase in stress on post-pelvic skeleton due to holding up body weight

6. Compromise in the equilibrium: the quadrupeds maintain a closed kinematic chain, whereas the biped bears an unstable open kinematic chain.

7. With upright stance, the circulatory system too has to undergo changes. In the biped, venous stasis in the lower limbs is not uncommon (varicosities). In the lower limbs, thrombo-angitis obliterans and anterior tibial syndrome are not uncommon circulatory system disorders.

8. The need for the oxygenated blood to travel vertically upwards to the brain also puts some strain on the arterial vessel walls causing aneurysms or rupture. Erect posture is theoretically at least, one of the causes of cerebral strokes.

9. Prolonged standing on feet could lead to compromise in the capillary circulation. In fact, in diabetics this is one of the causes for formation of foot ulcers.

10. The cervical vertebrae in the biped forms a stack of bones articulating with each other through facets placed both superiorly and inferiorly on their transverse processes. These joints are packed together with short ligaments that allow cervical muscles and beyond to produce flexion, extension and rotation. The vertical

disposition of the neck bones leads to a number of disorders in function and shape of the individual vertebrae. Osteoarthritic changes in hip and knee and formation of extra 'accommodative' uncovertebral (Luschka's) joints in the neck are often seen in older bipeds.

11. Pathological herniation of contents of the abdominal cavity is yet another problem associated with erect posture. The transfer of weight of organs and viscera to the pelvis poses a danger of herniation of a loop of intestine into the scrotal sac through the weight bearing and weakened inguinal openings. Moreover, the disappearance into vestiges of the pyramidalis, a muscle supporting the midline linea alba in man, also considerably weakens the anterior abdominal wall. Lumbar hernias are also exclusive to bipeds.

12. The development of varicocoeles, especially in the left testicular sac, is one of the known ill effects of bipedal stance.

13. Exposure of the face and front of the abdomen to injury; Blunt injuries to abdominal organs   is one of the pitfalls biped has to confront.

14, Formation of osteophytes or spurs on the calcaneum has been credited to prolonged strain and stress on this weight bearing tarsal.

11. 'March fractures' or stress fracture of the 3rd metatarsal has been attributed to occupational hazards in people who stay erect or standing for extended periods of time (soldiers)

12. Prolapses of intervertebral disc with compression of spinal nerves or collapse of the vertebra itself and conditions like scoliosis, lordosis and spondylitis are also often seen in the erect biped.

Walking gait consists of an alternating stance and swing of each leg; while the right leg is in swing the left leg is in stance and vice versa. In a normal gate the stance phase is about 62% while the swing phase only occurs in 38% of the time. Each of these two phases can be broken down further. The stance phase has five parts to it, the heel strike, foot flat, heel rise, push-off, and toe-off. During the push-off and toe-off stage the foot experiences the largest force, at nearly five times the body's weight; this force is placed on non-locked joints (from the pelvis down through the knee) and even the slightest sway of movement can disrupt the body's natural alignment.

The dramatic and substantial shift in the center of gravity engendered by change in posture forced modifications to and alterations in the structure, architecture and morphology of skeletal elements accompanied the shift from quadruped to biped posture and propulsion. Changes in the basi-sphenoid slope, The foramen magnum is located more inferiorly (Australopithicines have a more inferiorly placed foramen magnum) curvature and re-alignment in the vertebral column, changes in the position and shape of the pelvic girdle, angle of inclination and torsion in femur, change of structural and functional anatomy of the tibio-femoral (knee) joint, restructure in architecture and alignment of tarsi and alterations to foot biomechanics. Major morphological features diagnostic of bipedalism include: the presence of a bicondylar angle or valgus knee; a more inferiorly placed foramen magnum; the presence of a reduced or non-opposable big toe; a higher arch on the foot; a more posterior orientation of the anterior portion of the iliac blade; a relatively larger femoral head diameter; an increased femoral neck length; and a slightly larger and anteroposteriorly elongated condyles of the femur. Each of these features is a specific adaptation to address problems associated with bipedalism.

9

Tree climbing communities I

The human foot, though designed to bear weight and facilitate bipedal locomotion, also shows the combined effects of heredity and acquired lifestyle. Foot morphology is influenced by specialized occupation or specific usage's Adaptation in shape, and modifications in soft tissue and osteological components of the foot to large extent are dictated by kinesiological stresses and strains it is subject to. Functional biomechanics play a visually verifiable and metrically quantifiable anatomical remodeling of foot structure.

The role of evolution induced 'arch' formations in the foot in aiding early hominids adopt a terrestrial existence, abandoning forever, the arboreal life of his simian ancestors, is a landmark milestone in development of homo. The longitudinal arches of the foot, both medial and lateral play a vital and efficient role in easing human locomotion. The ligaments, joints, bones, muscles and soft tissue components of the foot, contribute in its own unique manner, in making man alone among his mammalian cousins, to have mastered the art of walking on hind imbs as units. The liberation of the forelimbs from its pithecoid compulsions for assisting locomotion has furthered hominid cerebration to discover its latent potential.

The question raised here is, are these time honored evolutionary anatomical features of the foot absolute? Can prolonged and sustained strain, induced by specific usages such as tree climbing, influence the foot structure to revert to its simian prototype? Are these changes, if any measurable? To answer some of these queries, we undertook a study of footprints of adult males drawn from communities that engage in tree climbing as an ancestral and hereditary calling.

The plantar footprint is a unique record of the weight bearing status is man. The print impress itself is a metrically assessable permanent database, which can be used to determine the functional efficiency of feet. Evaluation of the hemi-dome (hollowness) produced by the medial edge of the human foot, essentially the measurements of the components of the medial longitudinal arch should present us with data which can be compared and analyzed. In this paper we present our findings on the evaluation of booth feet of a hundred adult males, drawn at random from local communities that practice tree-climbing as a fulltime occupation. The results are compared with those collated from measurements in lay population of males drawn from the society at large.

An evaluation done on footprints both feet of a hundred adult male drawn at random, from local communities that practice tree-climbing as a fulltime occupation. Adult males from Thiyya, Idiga, Billava and Namdhari communities of three contiguous districts of the southwest coast of India formed the nidus for this study. The horizontal length, breadth and surface area of the hollow semilunar space in the prints were measured using Meyer's line as reference. The height of the medial arch was measured as a perpendicular drawn from the tuberosity of the navicular to the horizontal plane.

Field observations of the plantation industry, of palmyrah (toddy), areca and coconut were made to note the techniques of tree climbing used by professionals.

There is an obvious increase in all parameters, length, breadth, height and surface area in climbers compared to controls. It is also noted that the increase is directly proportional to the number of years of practice of the profession. However, oddly, the increase – trend gets arrested with climbers reaching three decades in experience.

Visual observations showed both feet in most climbers, especially those with a number of years of adherence to profession, had 'in-situ' partial inversion of foot. The hallux itself was invariably separated wide from the fellow toes (hallux valgus). Calcaneovarus and adduction deformations in both feet were also seen.

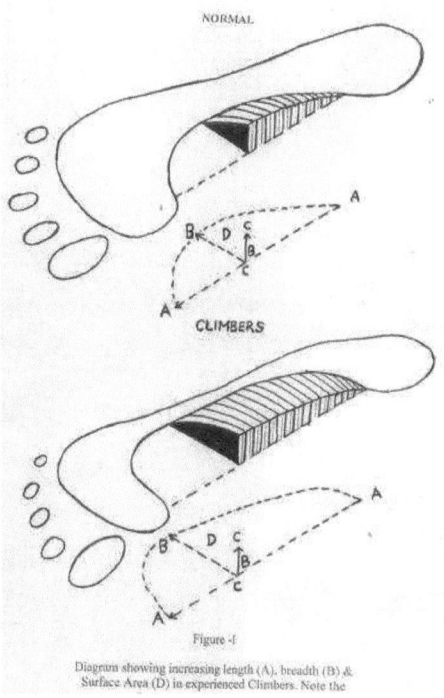

Figure -I

Diagram showing increasing length (A), breadth (B) &
Surface Area (D) in experienced Climbers. Note the

Fig: The height of the medial arch (C-C) rises with the number of years of climbing

35

Sociocultural compulsions make crops such as coconut, areca and palmyrah (toddy) economically viable for the planters. Sessional or regular plucking or tapping of palm produce requires specialized labor. This activity is traditionally carried out by isolated communities, the men-folk adeptly trained in the art of climbing trees rapidly. The communities engaged in this professional calling are distributed wherever palm is cultivated. The Idigas, Thiyya Namdhari and Billava have been tree climbers for generations and over the centuries.

The trees are scaled through a series of upward hops along the vertical face of the trunk, the exercise calling for flexion, abduction extension and lateral rotation of hip, flexion extension at knee, plantar and dosiflexion at ankle, inversion at the subtalar articulations and flexion at metatarsophalangeal and interphalangeal joints of the foot. To assist leverage, a 'rattan' loop is worn around the waist, which in turn is wound around the tree trunk. A similar loop worm across the ankles prevents the splaying of feet, keeping them approximated to the trunk surface at all times of ascent or descent. The climb induces tremendous gravitational strain on the tibiotalar and intertarsal joints, with each professional climber working about 4 hours a day, scaling 25-30 trees.

With sustained and prolonged strain at the joints, the foot undergoes permanent and quantifiable shape change. The enforced inversion, abuts on the osteo-myo-fascial bow of the medial longitudinal arch, which with time, shows an increase in length, breadth, surface area and height. These changes through quite rapid in the first few years of climbing, level off somewhat in the second decade of engagement, after which the dimensions once again show a spurt in all parameters. However, after three decades of climbing, the percentage values of increase drops for length, breadth and surface area, but continues to rise for height of arch.

The inference is that the foot dynamics and kinesiological exertions strain the factors maintaining the medial arch, the stress being overcome through a generalized augmentation in size and strength through intrinsic physiological compensatory counteractions. The failure of compensatory changes, with age and exposure (beyond 3 decades) leads to an arrest of these mechanisms, which now show a reduction in dimensions (and probably strength too.) The continued increase in arch height is mainly due to permanency of osteological changes in the foot architecture. The probable development of pressure induced epiphysis or bony spurs or buttresses in the tarsi through usage make the morphological adaptations in these bones permanent. The medial arch in experienced tree climbers is raised, not so much by the fascial inputs, but remains so by the rigidity of the deformed bony arch base.

It is also interesting to note that, accidental falls and fatalities that are recorded from time to time from groves, usually involve very experienced and old climbers. The mystery, why an experienced and highly skilled laborer should slip, may now be explained through our observations that, there is abrupt failure of arch resilience after 30 years climbing, evidenced in the rapid dip in dimensions of the hollowness.

In recent times, with falling economic returns from once cash – rich plantation industry, coupled with other factors – the rapid dwindling of able bodied men ready to stick to ancestral occupations (with availability of newer more lucrative and less strenuous avenues of income), and the palpable positive outcome of free education for all, along with constitutional guarantees to better opportunities for the tribal, backward and deprived segments of the populations it is very possible that decades hence, the complete lack of pluckers may drive the palm industry to seek totally mechanical means of cultivation. Studies such as this one may serve as retrievable records of the morphometrics of these 'dying' communities.

10

Tree climbing communities II

Coconut plantation crop is one of the agricultural activities in the southern part of India. Socio-cultural compulsions and regional culinary preferences have made coconut farming an economically viable for agriculturists. The maintenance of regular plucking and spraying of pesticides to coconut trees is which is done manually to a large extent, requires specialized laborers. This activity is traditionally carried out by the socio-economically backward communities, where men are trained in the art of climbing trees rapidly and plucking the coconuts or spraying pesticides.

These communities are distributed wherever coconut trees are cultivated in large numbers as coconut plantations. The trees are scaled through a series of upward hops along the vertical face of the tree trunk. The movements which call for flexion, abduction, extension and the lateral rotation of the hip, flexion and extension of the knees, plantar and dorsiflexion at the ankle, inversion at the subtalar joint, and flexion at metatarsophalangeal and interphalangeal joints of the foot, are required for climbing a vertically grown coconut tree. The arms flex, medially rotate and hold the tree trunk, while the body elevates to assist the leverage, a loop made of coir, is worn around the waist or between the palms, which in turn is wound around the tree trunk. A similar loop which is wound across the ankles, prevents the splaying of the feet, keeping them approximated to the trunk surface at all times of ascent or descent.

Climbing the coconut tree induces tremendous gravitational strain on the tibiotalar and the intertarsal joints, as each professional climber works about 4 hours a day, climbing 25-30 trees in a day. As India is in a transitional state in terms of the economic profile, an occupational research approach would balance between the understanding of the modern industrial exposures and the health risk of the traditional sectors like agriculture and plantations.

The technique of gripping the tree with both the hands and feet and thus pushing up the body to climb higher, results in intermittent pressure over the forearm, skin, palms and the soles.

The disabilities and the fatalities were very severe in the professional coconut tree climbers of rural southern India. Four coconut climbers who had fallen from trees died and two were disabled with paraplegia from the area of survey, according to the local daily newspapers. It is interesting to note that the accidental falls and fatalities usually involved the very experienced climbers. Colles, vertebral and maxillary fractures and tendocalcaneus lesions were few injuries that resulted due to fall from the coconut trees. It is felt that this was a more serious occupational hazard than the onboard slips and falls of flight attendants which preceded back pain. The climbers showed a decline in the Body Mass Index (BMI) and an increase in the rate of fall as the years of experience progressed.

11

The foot

The ankle-foot complex meets its diverse requirements through its 28 bones that form 25 component joints. The joints include, the proximal and distal tibiofibular joints, the ankle joint, subtalar joint, talonavicular and the calcaneocuboid joints, the five tarso metatarsal joints, five metatarsophalangeal joints and the nine interphalangeal joints. This complexity of the foot structure and the need to perform functions that has to undergo weight-bearing stresses will increase the frequency of ankle or foot problems. The approximate ranges of motion for adults in ankle joint are 20° of dorsiflexion and 30° of plantar flexion, from neutral. The range of motion in subtalar joint is around 15° of eversion and 35° of inversion

The ankle foot complex must meet both the stability demands and mobility demands in human body. The body requires a flexible foot to accommodate the variations in the external environment, a semi rigid foot that can act as a spring and lever arm for the push off during gait and a rigid foot to enable body weight to be carried with adequate stability The alterations of these functions in occupational demands like tree climbing can only be understood when studied in relation to the foot dynamics in gait cycle (the period of time for two steps in walking).In this paper we are presenting an unusual biomechanics of lower limb joints and its implications in professional coconut tree climbers of southern India These professionals are using this altered biomechanics 5-6 hours daily while doing their job, which lead to major anatomical and functional changes in their foot, which over a period of time lead to hazard of falling from trees

The gait cycle is divided into swing phase and stance phase. In swing phase, the foot swings forward to take another step. During the stance phase, the foot is in contact with the ground and Section can be divided into 5 steps in which the stages are heel strike, foot flat, midstance, heel off and toe off. The biomechanics of the foot are best explained by describing what happens to the foot during stance phase of the gait cycle. During heel strike to midstance the foot undergoes pronation. This movement allows the foot to adapt to uneven surfaces and it is during this phase that the foot acts as a shock absorber. As the body weight shifts forward, the feet begin to return to a neutral position in preparation to the heel off. During heel off, the foot begins to supinate. The foot bones, muscles and the plantar fascia act together to supinate to form a rigid lever. Abnormal amounts of pronation and supination leads to a variety of foot and leg problems. As in walking or climbing, the entire body acting as a closed kinematical chain, these abnormal biomechanics can create lower back, hip, knee, ankle and foot problems

Some researchers have argued that the last ancestor of human being was probably quite chimpanzee like including in its locomotion. But whether early hominins were adept tree climbers is not very clear. Kinematic data on vertical climbing in wild chimpanzees proves that they use large range of dorsiflexion ($45.5°\pm7.1°$) at the ankle joint while climbing trees. Most of their bodyweight is likely to be supported on a single highly dorsiflexed ankle at the stance phase during climbing, while the opposite foot is pushing off the substrate.

Although the coconut tree climbers use the similar vertical upward hops, most of them use ankle belt and grip both feet together while climbing. The maximum dorsiflexion during normal walking in modern humans is only $15°$-$20°$. Tree climbers had values of $33.3°\pm3.63°$ dorsiflexion while doing their routine occupation which is very high compared to the normal walking function of the human ankle joint.

Studies indicate that dorsiflexing the human ankle to 45° results in soft-tissue failure and severe injury, but our study reported no such soft tissue injuries in coconut tree climbers. But there is clear evidence that the increased range of dorsiflexion used for tree climbing will exert much pressure on the soft tissues around the ankle and foot which make them change or adapt to the occupation.

The anterior aspect of the distal tibia in climbing hominoids is predicted to be mediolaterally expanded as the contact area between the tibia and the talus shifts anteriorly during dorsiflexion. As invasive parameters are not included in our study, whether the tibia or any other skeleton of the foot complex adapted itself for this extreme dorsiflexion is unclear.

Literature indicates that from heel strike to the first 20% of stance phase the foot is in slight plantar flexion during normal walking. The foot begins to dorsiflex at this time and by 70% of stance phase the ankle dorsiflexion reaches from 7°to 14°.

In the final 30% of stance phase the foot plantar flexes again to prepare for the push off phase of walking and reaches a range of 14°-20°at push off. But, the vertical climbing in coconut tree requires initial dorsiflexion in stance phase (20°-36°) followed by plantar flexion (16°-51°),by push off. This extreme range also will affect the muscles supporting the osteoarchitecture of the foot.

Foot inversion at the subtalar and transverse tarsal joint are very important motion for positioning the sole of the foot against the vertical substrate during climbing bouts in arboreal primates. They have a bowed femur and an obliquely oriented tibia relative to the horizontal plane of the ankle joint.

43

This particular anatomy positions the knees lateral to the centre of gravity and places the free foot in an inverted set. But in contrast, the lower limbs are adapted for terrestrial bipedalism in humans. Humans have an obliquely oriented femur with a bicondylar angle and a tibia which is perpendicularly oriented relative to the plane of the ankle joint. Thus the sole of the human foot is directed plantar rather than medially when in neutral position.

This particular relationship in geometrics of the femur, tibia and foot in human has maladapted the human skeleton for arboreal locomotion. Even though the human foot is maladapted in its anatomy for dorsiflexion and inversion together in climbing as in arboreal primates, the coconut tree climbers of south India climb coconut trees with inversion and plantar flexion rather than dorsiflexion.

Arboreal primates safely and effectively climb trees as they are capable of extreme dorsiflexion at the ankle and inversion at the subtalar joints. The anatomical orientations of their lowerlimbs are suitable for arboreal habitat. Studies suggest that early hominid skeleton did not have adapted foot with extreme dorsiflexion and inversion so was not significant parts of their locomotor habits. A coconut tree climber who climbs more than 30 trees a day for 5-6 hours at a stretch is capable of extreme dorsiflexion, inversion and plantar flexion, similar to arboreal primates suggest that there is a probability for the skeletal adaptations in the foot.

The occupational hazard; falling from coconut tree while on job is seen in more experienced climbers. The altered biomechanics used by them in their profession might be the reason for it. As there is no published data regarding the biomechanics of coconut tree climbing, their occupational habits and probable osteological and functional atavism, we hope that this study provides the preliminary data for further studies.

12

The anatomy

The foot is merely a modified paddle: a spatulate dilatation developed at the distal ends of limbs: a series of levers acting through muscle activated multi-axial and multi-jointed skeletal elements. In every form of quadruped or biped, the foot is adapted to its particular mode of transportation, depending on the medium the foot is operated in – ground, water or air.

The foot and ankle complex is composed of twenty-eight irregular shaped bones making up twenty-five component synovial joints. It is compact, functionally efficient unit composed of osseous, fibrous, ligamentous, fascial and muscular components. The bony architecture is made of the tarsals: talus, calcaneus, navicular, cuboid, medial, intermediate and lateral cuneiforms and metatarsals, numbered I to V – articulating distally with the metatarsal heads are the proximal phalanges, which in turn articulate at their head ends with the intermediate phalanges, which in turn forms a joint with the distal phalanges. There are a total of 14 phalanges in a foot. There are three phalanges in each of the toes from II to V: The hallux, (I st. toe) carries only two, the proximal and distal. The bones of the foot are arranged along longitudinal two rays, the medial and lateral arches, each ray is composed of individual as well as shared bones: the talus, calcaneus, cuboid with the IVth. and Vth. metatarsal bones form the lateral longitudinal arch; the talus, calcaneus, navicular, cuneiforms, Ist., IInd. and IIIrd. metatarsals form the medial longitudinal arch.

Viewed from the plantar surface, the medial arch is higher than the lateral arch. The proximal ends of the arch bow is common, the calcaneus, while the distal end is formed by the head of the I st. metatarsal on the medial side and heads of the V th. metatarsal on the lateral side. The osseos architecture of the arches are maintained by numerous ligamentous that criss-cross bone to bone; the strongest among them being the plantar calcaneo-navicular (spring), the short and long plantar ligaments.

Besides the two named arches, other less obvious arches, the transverse arches too play an adjunct role in maintaining the functional integrity of the foot. The thick plantar skin and the plantar aponeurosis too help in support of the arches.

The muscles of the foot, both extrinsic and intrinsic provide an ideal three layered platform. Contraction of muscle masses and the tensing and easing of tendons as consequence play a major role in maintaining the arches: among these, more significant muscles are the peroneous longus and tibialis anterior et posterior.

The foot as a whole, can dorsiflex and plantar flex, the movements taking place at the tibio-talar and talo-fibular and inferior tibio-talar joints which together form a saddle to fit the surfaces and sides of the talus.

Within the foot itself, flexion and extension of metatarsals and digits, adduction, abduction of toes do take place through intrinsic joints. More significant movements, inversion and eversion take place through the sub-talar joint. A movement akin to pronation and supination can be performed by the foot.

The knee in man is a bicondylar joint endowed with the capability to 'lock' itself when fully extended. The capacity to lock gives man the potemtial to stand for extended periods on two legs without using energy; the muscles of the lower limb are not out to any stress as the weight of the individual is transmitted directly through the post pelvic skeletal elements when knee is locked. The limb can flex or extend and rotate to a small degree at its knee joint. The hip is a ball and socket, multiaxial joint allowing flexion, extension, adduction, abduction and rotation.

The femur is the longest and heaviest bone in the skeleton, built such for bearing and transmitting the body weight in biped erect posture and locomotion. The head and neck of the bone make an obtuse angle at their continuation as the upper end of the shaft. The usual angle is described to be ranged between 115 to 140°, with an average of 125°. The angle, wider at birth gradually diminishes with age. It is slighter lower in the female, due to the wider of the femoral shaft in the gender. The widened neck − shaft angularity facilitates the bone to swing clear of the pelvis during stories performed at the enarthrodial hip joint.

Analysis of the femora from Southern India, we present the results of our morphometrical consistently show that the angle of inclination is remarkably higher in populations and ethnic group that habitually use squatting as a posture of ease and preferred comfort from very early age.

The angle of inclination ranged from a low of 130° to a high of 158° in this study, with the mean angle being 146°. It was also observed that the bones showed the distinctive squatting facet on their lower end and that the length of the femoral neck was foreshortened in every specimen.

The consistent finding of a significant 10% to 15% increase in neck − shaft angulation in every bone measured leads us to believe that reversal of roles for weight bearing from the superior surface of the femoral head to the its inferior surface engendered by habitual squatting plays a major role induces change in trabecular weight - transmission patterns, which in turn re-morphs the angle of inclination more obtusely.

Non metric post pelvic skeletal changes have been reported periodically. These in the main, in the lower limbs, are those caused by the socio – cultural anthropological postural preference, squatting, especially in sub – continental Asians. Among the permanent impressions formed in the post pelvic osseous elements are facets found on the upper surface of talar neck, lower anterior end of tibia and both ends of the femur.

That squatting formed an integral part of daily life in the specimens studied is confirmed by that fact that all the femora were of local origin, and each of them displayed the tell tale squatting facet on their lower end, just below the adductor tubercle over – riding the medical femoral condyle.

This wide variation in the angle of inclination in femora and the correlation of the increase to postnatal influences induced by socially generated physical adaptations in ethnic populations. The angle deformation may play an important role as an identity marker for geographical assignment of skeletal remains, especially during forensic investigations following mass disasters.

13

Remote skeletal effects: I

Much has been studied and reported on the skeletal changes as consequence of bipedal stance and gait, yet most of the research output concentrates on changes observed in the pelvic and post-pelvic skeletal elements. Yet, the bony framework functions as a single unit, with individual mobile and fixed parts. It is reasonable to infer that any change in any one element or part of the lower limb should translate or find echo in changes in size, function or shape of more distal parts of the skeleton. In fact almost every pre-pelvic part of the biped skeleton refelect adap[tiove alterations to their anatomy as consequence of hind-limbs taking over the weight bearing and locomotor functions.

The skull, cranium, vertebral column, upper limb and sacrum show changes in the biped.

The human skull is unique in that it bears a number of bones that are hollow within. These pockets called sinuses are predominantly positioned in and around the anterior half of the skull, and are known as paranasal air sinuses. The maxillary, frontal (paired) the sphenoidal and ethmoidal (unpaired) sinuses lie within the maxillae, frontal, ethmoid and sphenoid bones.

Much time and space has been taken up by physical anthropologists and human biologist in debating and discussing the reason for presence and roles played by air sinuses in the human skull.

Among the many theories proposed, the few that are accepted as reasonably sound are:

1. The sinuses lighten the skull weight

2. The sinuses warm inhaled air

3. The sinuses provide resonance to human voice

4. Provide protection

5. Play a role in humidifying inhaled air.

The skull is a heavy unit of bones supported and held up merely through two small articular facets on the atlas (1st cervical) vertebra. It is quite interesting to observe that such a massive weight contained in the by the skull, a weight made up by bones, tissues, muscle mass, glands, vessels, meninges and the brain, has just a pair of supports – the two atlanto-occipital joints.

It has been observed that in some animals, using mouth / nose / tail as accruements that can aid or initiate movement: yet it would seem strange to learn that the ability use mouth parts are adjuncts to movement. In fact as described elsewhere it is indeed so. The description of the atavistic oro-facial reflex is example of how the mouth, involuntarily, plays a role.

Years of observation over large populations have reinforced my surmise that a hitherto unnoticed facial reaction is a legacy of atavism. The higher the degree of digital dexterity involved in the performance of manual tasks, the more striking is the involuntary reaction of orofacial muscles to the level of concentration the task requires. Watch a volunteer thread a needle; the individual either purses his lips, or contorts his mouth, or licks his lips, or bites his tongue tip; An orofacial-lingual response to manual work?

As this is a very widespread and universally human response, it must have either a functional or atavistic basis, if not so. In quadrupeds, simians specially, the mouth or its component parts, the teeth, lips or tongue, are used as adjuncts to bimanual work. The use of oral appendages as adjunct aids in performance of manual tasks certainly makes, tearing, ripping, or carrying food or material.

Is the human involuntary reaction of facial grimace, twitch, wetting, or clenching the jaw, a physiological atavistic trait carried over into the higher mammal? How does the contraction of orbicularis oris or the action of genioglossus muscle influence the performance of task at 'hand'?.

There is no obvious correlation or between the disparate muscular masses, the direct use of the hand lumbricals to perform concentrated manual chore, and the simultaneous, but, indirect oro-facial muscular action of the mouth and tongue. The muscle groups involved (in hand and of mouth) are neither contiguous nor congruous or complementary, yet they occur together.

It is inferred that the digito-oro-facial-lingual response to performance of manual work requiring concentrated effort is an un-reported evolutionary vestige and a classic, but odd, non-anatomical vestige of atavism.

Of similar genre is the tripping over or falling seen in bipeds. The kinetics of biped gait makes the human unstable. The tendency to fall is very inherent to movement on two supports (legs). But observe the fall: it is always forwards – almost never backwards. Whenever a man trips, he stumbles forwards – the reflex direction of fall enables him to quickly support his falling weight on his outstretched hands (forelimbs). This protective reflex mechanism is inborn.

Observing an infant on the move is perhaps the closest one can see the inherent 'quadruped' factors that are inbuilt. Firstly, a baby needs to be supported at its head end when being carried or lifted; the head wobbles when unsupported.

Second, the mandible has no teeth. Third, sinuses are not seen as they are yet to develop. The first and second factors demonstrate that the head is too heavy for the infantile supports to hold it up, even without the additional weight of teeth or the lightening of weight through air sinuses.

Observe also that in the infant, the mandible is small and bears no teeth and the sinuses are undeveloped. Both these appear at a later stage of childhood, raising the total weight of the anterior and middle third of the head.

To support the head in upright posture, the foramen magnum and its adjacent basi-occipital articular facets had to migrate forwards and downwards at reach right to the bottom of the skull. The human head weighs around 3.5 to 4.5 kilograms. The entire cranial unit along with its suspended mandible bears down on the atlanto-occipital joints to be held up, extend, flex or rotate.

As the supporting pillars formed by the cervical vertebrae are (as viewed from the norma lateralis) is positioned more towards the posterior third of the skull base, every part of the skull along with the mandible lies in front (anterior) to the weight supporting joints.

Imagine the unit as simply osseous, without muscular, membranous (atlantooccipetal) or ligamentous attachments – the entire head would tilt forwards (flex). The long arm of the lever lies anterior to the fulcrum (atlanto-occipital joint); the short arm extends posteriorly. Obviously there is an extra weight in the front of the fulcrum, forcing the skull of nod forward (flex) by itself in situ. To counter the mechanical skew, one needs to hinge (slide) the skull backwards to maintain it at even keel in a horizontal plane. The parity is restored only when muscles and ligaments counteract and overcome the skewed weight ratios. Here is where one observes the multitude of muscle masses attached (splenius capitis, semispinalis capitis along with muscles in the suboccipetal area) to the squamous part of the external occipital crest, which itself provides mooring to the ligamentum nuchae, another major factor maintaining head leveling. Note that all these muscles lie behind the atlanto-occipital joints – their contraction producing extension of neck. Yet another muscle, the sternocliedomastid, attached above to the mastoid process and below to the clavicle and sternum, crosses the joint above downwards obliquely. Its contraction too extends the head. The trapezius, along with the ligaments and stylohyoid, stylomandibular, sternohyoid and the strap muscles that attach to hyoid play accessory roles in the extension and maintenance of balance of the cranium / head.

Taking a new look at within the skull, the posterior cranial fossa in the biped is situated a step lower than the middle fossa, bringing its content the cerebellum, to lie lower than the temporal and occipital lobes of the cerebrum. In quadrupeds the cerebellum lies approximately at the same level (or slightly below) the cerebral hemispheres. The shift in position of the hindbrain from behind the forebrain to below it and the adjunct displacement of the posterior cranial fossa to a level lower than in the quadruped skull, reduces the forebrain to hindbrain angulation, enabling the head to be held vertically up the vertebral column without pressurizing, stressing or straining the spinal cord.

The entire relocation of the osseous and nervous components in the posterior third of the head demonstrates that in needing to hold the head vertically up at erect posture and in bipedal gait, the shift in weight of the cerebellum to its completely new position, infero-posterior to both, the cerebrum and the atlanto-occipital joints, raises the weight of the short arm of the lever (fulcrum at the joint). The key postural reflex or major site of the kinesthetic sense is located at the atlanto The entire relocation of the osseous and nervous components in the posterior third of the head demonstrates that in needing to hold the head vertically up at erect posture and in bipedal gait, the shift in weight of the cerebellum to its completely new position, infero-posterior to both, the cerebrum and the atlanto-occipital joints, raises the weight of the short arm of the lever (fulcrum at the joint). The key postural reflex or major site of the kinesthetic sense is located at the atlanto - occipital area

This is done by 'emptying' (hollowing) some bones that form the face and middle third of the skull. The maxillae, the frontals, the ethmoid and sphenoid are filled with air pockets – the paranasal air sinuses.

Now that the evolutionary scheme of things re-morph the skull and relocate its contents to aid erect posture, bringing more 'weight' posterior to the atlanto-occipital joints, it also augments the mechanical skewing of advantage due to of lever systems functioning at the joints by reducing the weight in the long arm of the lever, the anterior third of the skull.

To sum up, in going bipedal, the remote skeletal changes taking place are:

a. The deepening and level lowering of the posterior cranial fossa

b. Shifting of the cerebellum from behind the posterior part cerebrum to below it. In effect, the cerebrum, cerebellum attempt to stack themselves one over another, instead of one behind another (as is in quadrupeds) to enable weight transmission along a vertical axis

c. Repositioning the occipital opening for the hind brain, the foramen magnum to its new antero-inferior location

d. Reshaping the slope of the basi-sphenoid (the clivus) to a steeper plane.

e. Tethering, mooring and holding the posterior third of the skull through ligaments and muscles- ligamentum nuchae and sternocliedomastoid along with a number of localized short muscles and ligaments in the suboccipital region. The taut atlantooccipital membrane too functions as a tether.

f. Reducing the weight in the anterior half / third of the head and skull by hollowing out bony matter from sphenoid, ethmoid, maximale and frontals to form sinuses.

The mandible is suspended from the base of the skull through its moor, the tempero-mandibular joint. Its entire weight is borne by the skull in the biped. In the light of the discussion earlier on uneven distribution of weight of head along the horizontal axis with reference to the lever mechanism operating at atlantooccipital joints, the mandible along with its dentition augments the load on the anterior arm of the lever. Despite compensatory mechanisms to counter the excess weight anteriorly (through repositioning of cerebellum and hindbrain and guy-wire like supports through occipital muscles), the anterior position of the skull too divests itself of some weight by emptying its sinuses of osseous tissue. The mandible itself is light at birth (as related to head weight) increasing in dimension and weight as age advances. In a fully developed adult mandible a full complement of teeth adds to the total weight of the bone.

The question is can the bone itself try something different to shed weight as a part compensation to restoration of lopsided weight ratio anteriorly and along the horizontal axis passing through the fulcrum (atlanto-occipital joints)? In early man, just trying out a few strides of bipedal gait, the mandible was a massive chewing unit: with time and refinement in an overall reduction in mandibular body size and dentition in weight of the jaw evolved simultaneously. The alveolar ridge itself shortened in length crowding out space for growth of the third molars. The impaction of the growing molar is one of the more common afflictions seen by the dental surgeon.

Herein I may add that the mysterious (but uncommon) presence of the 'Stafne's cyst' in the ramus of the mandible – considered by some to be an embryonic relic- could in some probability be a natural event in evolutionary biology to reduce the weight of the mandible itself.

Similar too, is the fate the maxillary third molar: it too finds itself edged out by the reduction in space available on the alveolar margin. One of the theories is that the wisdom teeth are vestigial third molars that used to help human ancestors in grinding down plant tissue. While possibly true, the more rational inference could be that the molars were lost as price paid for by man for going erect and biped.

Add the weights of the four molar teeth to that of weight lost by absence of osseous matter from the sinuses to overall reduction in body size and weight of mandible and maxilla – and you end up with a fairly large reduction in total weight in the anterior part of the head.

14

Remote skeletal effects: II

The vertebral column is made of a series of irregular bones, each atop another. The cranial end of the column is the atlas and the caudal end in formed by the fifth lumbar vertebra resting on the sacrum. Each vertebra is separated from its partner by the inter-vertebral disc, a non osseous fibro-cartilaginous cushion.

Observing the layout and architecture of the bony spine, one is struck by its similarity to a tree trunk. The column widens, much like a tree's buttresses, the last vertebra in the lumbar series being the widest. It is clearly obvious that to bear the weight of the head, neck, thorax and abdomen and their contents, the column has to become broader as it gathers size and substance t bear extra weight. In man, the widening is reinforced by the erect posture he has taken.

The sacrum, a single unit made of unionized individual sacral vertebrae, is a curved plate of bone shaped like a wedge. Its wide flanges, the alae and body provide attachment to numerous strong ligaments and muscles that firmly tether it to the pelvis girdle and beyond. The sacrum itself is according some, a 'keystone' element helping to 'fix' the bones around the girdle. Others dispute this claiming the sacrum does not play any key role as it is situated in a manner that, without mooring, it should slide / slip forwards.

Whatever the argument, it is clear that all the weight of the head and torso are transmitted to the sacrum and through its lateral surface onto the pelvic bones and thereon to the lower limbs.

The transmission of weight along the vertical axis in the erect postured does often lead to prolapsed of disc with compression of spinal nerves or collapse of the vertebra itself: conditions such as scoliosis and spondylitis are also caused by changeover to biped posture and locomotion.

Elbow: Widening of pelvic brim, in turn influences the 'carrying angle' of the upper limb. The medial condyle of the humerus lies at a lower level than in the male, reducing the outer angle at the elbow. This shift in angulation is not seen in the quadruped. Moreover, the broadening of the pelvis, as whole, also creates the 'pre-auricular sulcus' in the female sacrum.

Ribs & thorax: The antero-posterior diameter of the bony thoracic cavity is reduced at the cost of transverse diameter in the erect. The downward tug of visceral abdominal contents probably influence the change of the diameters in the biped thorax

Besides the above mentioned, the sacroiliac (to an extent), intervertebral and other axial joints play a role in maintenance to posture and performance of bipedal gait. The pelvis is turned and tilts forwards in the biped, transferring weight anteriorly: in the female, the pelvis widens during maturity, allowing the inlet to accommodate for parturition.

15

Theories & hypotheses

Among the many theories and hypotheses proposed on the possible reasons for an advanced species of pan going biped to evolve into homo are the following. Evolutionary biologists and anthropologists despite heated debates and disagreements favoring one or the other, however concede that there could be more than one specific cause for the shift from a predominantly quadruped gait to a bipedal one. A combination of theories makes more sense.

Going through the list one readily observes that each one of them appears as rational as another, yet one is left with a lurking suspicion that there could perhaps be more, many more, as yet un-discovered and un-described scenarios that could have engendered two-legged gait and erect stance

Watching-out Hypothesis: Many animals do stand up on two hind legs for better view of surroundings. It is fairly common among meercats and bears.

Freeing of the Hands Hypothesis: Liberating two out of four limbs from burden of locomotion for other uses.

Throwing Hypothesis: An extension of the previous theory

Infant Carrying Hypothesis: The human neonate is a helpless being. Toting a baby is a fine art – many animals use their mouth, others cradle their newborns and infants on the belly (and holding them in place using a foreleg) or on the back if little older.

Reaching for Food / Carrying Food Hypothesis: Reaching for food sources at higher levels, gathering them in the arms or hands could have lead to biped positioning

Display Hypothesis: Posturing for threat display, raising size of appearance through standing up. Phallic display as sexual come-on is an extension of this hypothesis.

Orthograde Scrambling Hypothesis: Bipedal gait could have been a part and parcel of a series of movements that the primate used on a regular basis (orangutan) but perfected in the later pan,

Scavenging Hypothesis: Is, at best, an extension of the carrying hypothesis.

Aquatic Ancestor Hypothesis: A controversial theory that proposes that terrestrial movement was triggered by the migration of an aquatic ape that had to use legs to that up or move

Wading Hypotheses: Here it is postulated that the some australopithecines when wading through water, had to stand up or walk. Feeding off aquatic environs too needed an upright stance to keep the torso, head and neck above water level.

Thermoregulation Hypothesis: The movement across vast shade-less savannahs through scorching sun could have made the ape stand upright to reduce exposure to solar heat.

Climbing Hypothesis: Some biologists believe that the rugged savannah terrain made the later quadruped apes to use forelimbs to hold on to fixed objects to scale steep slopes and inclines.

Mounting hypothesis: The topic on origins of erect (orthograde) stance and bipedal gait has provided evolutionary biologists   much material for discussion, debate and postulations. Over the years, a number of hypotheses have been proposed, each justifying its own rationale and logic for acceptance. To this fairly exhaustive list of theories, I let me add another: the sexual 'mounting'.

Nearly every quadruped 'mounts' its mate during copulation. The stance facilitating penetration, serves to transfer a major portion of the body weight in the male, to its hind legs. However, animals (mammals) mate or are receptive to mating only when female is in oestrus, a periodic cyclical physiological event. As such, mating activity is time specific and limited, yet, when considering that in higher primates, chimpanzees - bonobos in particular, sexual activity is continuous having no specific relationship to oestrus, this 'mounting as predecessor to erect posture and biped gait' theory makes more sense.

Bonobo chimpanzees are observed to 'mount' regularly, routinely and almost non-stop, the behavior is usually a 'simulated' copulatory action, said to reinforce social bonding within the primate groups. The frantic mounting requiring standing or supporting body weight on lower limbs probably engendered extension of bipedal weight support into erect posturing and thence, also to striding. Remarkably in bonobos even females mount each other often, showing that standing up on hind limbs is an activity spanning the gender gap.

More significantly, bonobos are possibly the closest 'relative' of the hominid, sharing around 99% of their genetic make-up. It is eminently logical and rational to postulate that the prelude to erect posture and biped gait was an offshoot of the frequent and repetitive acts of 'mounting' practiced by both sexes of man's closest surviving ancestor, the chimpanzee.

The body weight bearing on the lower limbs as part of mounting activity, not only strengthened the limbs, but possibly triggered the process of realigning of post-pelvic musculature, especially in the gluteal, back of thigh hamstring) and back of leg (tendocalcaneus) and alterations in skeletal architecture of the pelvis, knee and foot.

Other theories and hypotheses that cross my mind are presented here: It is possible too that the surface heat on terrain directly exposed to a scorching sun could have made quadrupedal gait stressful and agonizing – could the bipedal stride have evolved as a counter to reducing surface area of anatomy directly in contact with a heated earth? Desert reptiles such as sidewinder snakes actually sidle across the hot dunes raising the body as do some lizards which stand on three legs at a time, instead of on four. Some can actually scamper rapidly on two hind legs too when things get too hot! (pardon the pun) !

Observe how the modern mother tugs and yanks her reluctant toddler down the shopping mall's aisle. She actually drags him holding his hand in hers; The youngster now held up awkwardly, struggles to find his feet and willingly or not, scrambles to his feet and scampers with her matching her pace, step by step.......on two legs. The example here illustrates what might well have been true 4 million years ago.

Imagine an ape, an early biped and female, unable to carry its babe physically due to the infant's increasing weight, forcing him to move alongside her, part dragging it part supporting its, enabling it through trial, error, scrape and slip, helping it to steady itself on its two baby legs; A small baby step then...but what a mighty leap for the hominid.

When on the move, the newborn in simians and apes cling onto their mother's coat, belly or are held close to chest by the mother's supporting arm. Imagine when the tiny one crosses a certain weight. Then, either use four legs to keep up with mum, or try emulate her when she is walking on two by holding on to her hand or her hip /leg.

So let us add two more possible scenarios that spawned bipedalism.

(a) Walking the infant alongside its mother, who by extending support to its two legged stance and stride, schools it to mastery over the two legged gait

(b) Scorched terrain for the quadruped could have forced it to use, on occasion, three legs or even two, to keep the heat off its paws. Dessert reptiles, lizards, do lift one or two legs off the hot dunes and sands to avoid getting seared. Probably the pioneer biped did – it used its hndlegs to support itself, keeping its forelimb paws off the searing hot ground.

16

The liberated forelimb

It is one of the mysteries: why did some life forms like birds who mastered bipedal gait quite early in the evolutionary time scale not use their free forelimbs for uses other than for flying? The huge advantage the liberation from using the front legs for quadruped gait, acquired by the birds, quite inexplicably was not exploited to its hilt; the forelimb modified into wings was used almost wholly by the animal to fly – locomotion through a non-terrestrial medium – air.

A few species of birds do put their winged forelimbs to other uses, but none do so ass efficiently, intelligently or advantageously as the hominines. The lapwing uses when occasion demands its wings to protect its clutch as do some other species that spread their wings to shade their young from a directly overhead sun. It is to be noted here that the earliest birds could use a clawed wing to climb tree trunks. Even today, one species retains that talent in its infancy – the hoatzin (*Opisthocomus hoazin*)

A few other birds spread their wings to appear larger to scare foes. Apart from an odd example here and there, birds in the main, use their forelimbs in flight.

Monkeys and apes, quadruped as they are, occasionally free their forelimbs from functioning as merely appendages helping locomotion. Capuchin monkeys crack nuts and almost all simians groom each other using their paws. Chimpanzees are known to use stones and crude implements to smash or toss objects. Gorillas use their front limbs to beat their chest or make their 'nests'.

The above examples notwithstanding, only in the hominid do we observe an extensive and wide application of the potential, prowess and power made available by the free upper limb. One debate stands out here: how did the missing link or early biped suddenly become adept in using hands?

For much of the answer, we have to look beyond the pelvis and lower limb. The upper limb may well be the key to the riddle. With the evolution of the hand and fingers into useful and adaptable instruments, circumstances changed the way the thumb (pollex) evolved. The human pollex is almost exclusive in that it possesses a first carpometacarpal joint which is a 'saddle'. The wide range of movements has another unique articulation, the opposability of the thumb. Thumb – index opposition as contrasted with thumb-index 'apposition' was the final frontier in the refinement of the hand into an instrument of versatility. With this articular refinement, an explosion in cerebral powers followed; the need to conjure or create ways and means in exploiting the potential and function of the newly developed edge gave much gist to thinking and thought processing. The boost in capacity and capability of the brain in turn led to the australopithecine turning into hominids.

The swinging arms:

Bipedal gait is odd in that despite the forelimbs being completely excluded from the burden of carrying weight or helping in locomotion, they do form an integral part of the biped's movement cycle. Observe how the free upper limbs swing forwards and backwards with every stride the lower limbs take. Each upper limb alternates its 'to and fro' sortie in synch with its contralateral lower limb counterpart.

Now, picture the scene with the same biped hominid walking forwards, but with his body flexed forwards at his hip joints and palms at ground level. The gait now so resembles a typical quadruped's; very much like a dog or cat walking on all four limbs, alternating one forelimb of one side with the hind limb of the other.

References & Bibliography

1.Arunachalam Kumar (2012) Knuckle walking as prelude to hominin bipedality or acquired mechanism to protect fingertips? Nitte University Journal of Health Science, 2 (2): 41-42

2.George BM, Muddanna SR, Arunachalam Kumar, 2013; Biomechanics of climbing coconut trees and its implications in ankle-foot morphology, Journal of Clinical & Diagnostic Research, Vol.7, No.5, 789-793

3.Arunachalam Kumar, 2013; Cranio-caudal displacement of propulsive accruements: evolutionary markers? Journal of Biological Sciences, Vol.6 (1) 30-31

4.George BM, Arunachalam Kumar, Muddanna SR, 2013; Foot Deformations in Coconut Tree Climbers of South India, Nitte University Journal of Health Science, Vol.3 (1) 45 – 51

5.Stafne, EC. Bone cavities situated near the angle of the mandible, JADA 1942; 29:1969–197

6.Johnson, George B. "Evidence for Evolution". Txtwriter Inc., 8 Jun 2006

7.George BM, Muddanna SR, Arunachalam Kumar, 2013; Biomechanics of climbing coconut trees and its implications in ankle-foot morphology, Journal of Clinical & Diagnostic Research, Vol.7, No.5, 789-793

8.Arunachalam Kumar, 2013; Hopping in Birds: is The Choice of Gait Influenced by Cervical Mobility and Field of Vision? Nitte University Journal of Health Science, Vol.3 (1) 56 - 58

9.Vishal K., Vinay K.V., Remya K., Arunachalam Kumar & Shishir K, 2012; High Sacral Hiatus with Non Fusion of Lamina of First Sacral Vertebrae: A Case Report, Nitte University Journal of Health Science, Vol.2 (4)

10.Carsten Niemitz (2010), The evolution of the upright posture and gait—a review and a new synthesis, Naturwissenschaften., 97 (3): 241–263

11.Remya K, Arunachalam Kumar & Vishal K, 2012; The unco-vertebral joints of Luschka, Nitte University Journal of Health Science, Vol.2, No.4

12.Arunachalam Kumar, 2012, Knuckle-walking: prelude to hominin bipedality or acquired mechanism to protect fingertips? Nitte University Journal of Health Science Vol.2, No.2

13.Bincy M. George, Muddanna SR, Arunachalam Kumar, Niveditha S, JS D'Souza, 2012; Health of coconut tree climbers of rural south India - Medical emergencies, body mass index and occupational marks- a quantitative and survey study; Journal of Diagnostic and Clinical Research Vol. 6 (1) pp 57- 60

14.Arunachalam Kumar; An overview on evolution of human erect posture, bipedal mobility and gait, RGUHS Journal of Medical Sciences 1: 3: 35-41, 2011

15.Arunachalam Kumar, The Gondwanaland crescent as home to hominid gene pool, Philosophy of evolution, Transcience Transactions Vol.1, Yash Publications, Bikaner, 2010

16.Bhat PS & Arunachalam Kumar; The medial longitudinal arch in tree climbing communities, Scientific Medicine 1 (2) 2009

17.Ganesh KC, Arunachalam Kumar et al; Morphology of lacrimal sac and lacrimal duct in cadaver, Bratislava Medical Journal, 110 (11) 740-743, 2009

18.Vivek Y, Bhoppi R, Arunachalam Kumar et al, The femoral neck-shaft angle in squatters, Ind. J. Forensic Med. Toxic., 3; 1: 2009

19.Ranade A, Prabhu LV & Arunachalam Kumar, Morphometric study of the tibial collateral ligament, International Journal of Morphology, 24 (4) 677-678, 2006

20.Arunachalam Kumar & Kumar JC; Atavistic Orofacial Response to Manually Dexterous Activity, Medical Hypotheses, Vol. 65: 161, 2005

21.Arunachalam Kumar; Non-metric Analysis of Post-cranial Skeleton, Indian Journal of Forensic Medicine & Toxicology Vol. 14 (2) No 29, 1997

22.Arunachalam Kumar & Pai ML; Foramen Magnum Index for Sexing Adult Indian CraniaAnatomical Adjuncts, Vol. 1 No. 7, 1988

23.Arunachalam Kumar & Koranne SP; Squatting Facet on Femora in the West Coastal Indian Population, Forensic Science International, Vol. 21 No. 2, 19, 1983

24.Arunachalam Kumar; An Osteological Clue to Bipedalism; Human Races Monthly, Vol.1, No. 9, 2002

25.Arunachalam Kumar; A Tear Shed, Again, for Bipedalism; Human Races Monthly, Vol.1, No. 9, 2002

26.Arunachalam Kumar; Shedding a Tear for Bipedalism; Human Races Monthly, Vol. 1, No. 9, 2002

27.Arunachalam Kumar; The Index digit rotation and opposition evolution; Human Races Monthly, Vol. 1, No.9, 2002

28.Arunachalam Kumar; Hominid Fossils in India: Some Predictions; Human Races Monthly, Vol. 1, No. 9, 2002

29.Arunachalam Kumar; Brachiation 'one small step' for mankind? Human Races Monthly, Vol. 1, No. 9, 2002

30.Arunachalam Kumar; 'The Kumar Hypothesis' on Hominid Fossil Finds in India; Human Races Monthly, Vol. 1, No. 9, 2002

32.Arunachalam Kumar; Fossil Finds in India: Early Hominids; Human Races Monthly, Vol. 1, No. 9, 2002

33.Arunachalam Kumar; The why of knuckle walking; http://network.nature.com/groups/transcience/forum/topics/5454

34.Arunachalam Kumar; Are squatting facets more than osteological oddities? http://network.nature.com/groups/transcience/forum/topics/5450

35.Arunachalam Kumar; Cranio-caudal shift in locomotor biomechanisms during evolution http://network.nature.com/groups/transcience/forum/topics/5395

36.Arunachalam Kumar; Kumar's gene saturation theory Part I http://network.nature.com/groups/transcience/forum/topics/5277

37.Arunachalam Kumar; Kumar's gene saturation theory: chaos: Part II http://network.nature.com/groups/transcience/forum/topics/5365

38.Arunachalam Kumar; A look at mass extinction; http://network.nature.com/groups/transcience/forum/topics/54981

39.Arunachalam Kumar; Shedding a tear for bipedalism Parts I & II; http://network.nature.com/groups/transcience/forum/topics/5451

40.Arunachalam Kumar; Erect posture: the handicaps of bipedalism; CDE, Indian Dental Association, DK Branch, Mangalore, 2011

41.Bincy MG, Arunachalam Kumar & Muddanna SR, 2011; Occupational adaptations in plantar contact areas of coconut climbers of south India, International Conference on Occupation Health, Bangkok

42.Bincy MG, Arunachalam Kumar & Mudanna SR, 2010; Quantifiable anatomical changes in professional coconut tree-climbers of South India: Is there atavism. National Conference, ASI, Pune

43.Kumar J C & Arunachalam Kumar; Chaotic Plantar Weight Distribution in Bipeds; National Conference, A.S.I., Hyderabad, 2004

44.Nayak S, Bhat S & Arunachalam Kumar; Analysis of Plantar Prints in Tree-climbing Communities; National Conference, A.S.I., Hyderabad, 2004

45.Oberoi DV, Arunachalam Kumar, Kumar JC., ; Non-chaotic weight-bearing foci & diabetic foot ulceration? ; International Conference on Endocrinology. Jaipur;2005.

46.Oberoi DV, Kumar JC & Arunachalam Kumar, 2006; Non chaotic weight bearing foci and diabetic foot ulceration; PG Medical Conference, Annamalai University

47.Arunachalam Kumar; Fossil Finds in India: Early Hominids; Human Races Monthly, Vol. 1, No. 9, 2002

48.Prabhu L V & Arunachalam Kumar; The Functional Anatomy of the Lacrimal Sac: A Reassessment; 48th A.S.I. National Conference, Manipal, 2001

49.Anuradha & Arunachalam Kumar; Observations on the Tibial Collateral Ligament; 46th. A.S.I. National Conference, Karad, MH 1998

50.Savita S & Arunachalam Kumar; The Thumb-Index Complex Biomechanics in Opposition; XIV Conference of Indian Society of Hand Surgeons, Manipal, 1990

51.Savita S & Arunachalam Kumar; The Tibial Collateral Ligament: Morphology & VariationsXIC State Conference, Karnataka Orthopaedics Society, Mangalore, 1990

52.Rao A & Arunachalam Kumar; Opposition Biomechanics: A Community Study; National Conference on Biomedical Engineering, Manipal, 1998

53.Savita S & Arunachalam Kumar; The Unco-vertebral Joints of Luschka; XVI State Conference, Karnataka Orthopaedic Association, Belgaum, 1993

54.Arunachalam Kumar; Developmental defects of the Skeletal System; South Kanara Homoeopaths Association Seminar, Mangalore, 1985

55.Das R, Pai ML & Arunachalam Kumar; Foramen Magnum Index for Sexing Adult Indian Crania; 1st World Conference of Forensic Medicine & Toxicology, Bhopal, 1984

56.Arunachalam Kumar & Pai ML; Greater Sciatic Notch Angle: An Additional Parameter for Sexing Adult Hip Bones, IV National Conference, Indian Academy of Forensic Science, Hyderabad, 1981

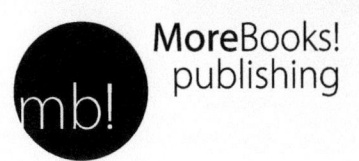
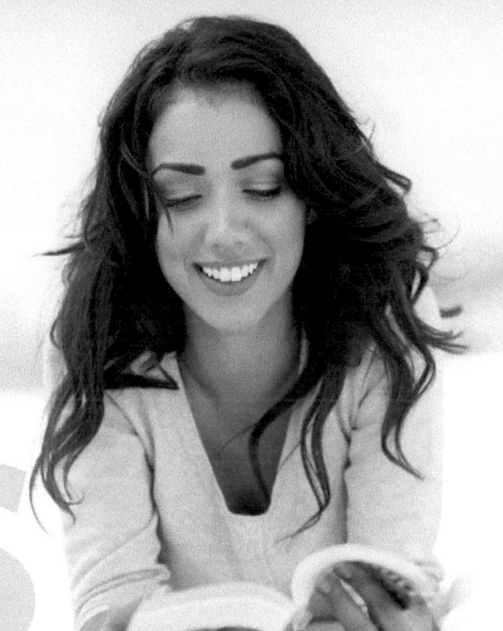
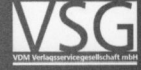

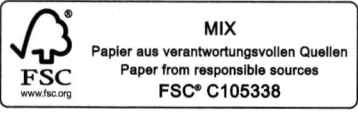